Movies On Paper Studio

Presents

Cancer Survival Museum

Title Page for: **Cancer Survival Museum**

This self -help novel was created By: Dionne L. Fields

Dionne L. Fields also made other contributions to this book title.

Illustrated

Photograph

Proofread

Editorial

Written

By Dionne Fields

1. Fields, Dionne. -Business 2.Woman Business Owner 3.African-American Author Patients-United States-Biography. 4. Publisher and Entrepreneur.5. Movies On Paper Studio.
6.Fields, Rain. 7. Ideas On Paper, 8. Sitcoms On Paper, Episode 1 and 10. Episode 2.

Book Title: Cancer Survival Museum

ISBM 978-1507736128
ISBM 10-1507736126

Movies on Paper Studio **NonFiction** Children's Book Collection.

1.Rain's 1st Christmas,
2.Actor Rain,
3. Inventor Rain,
4. Super Model Rain,
5.God's Child One
6.Recording Artist Rain,
7.Surfboarder Rain
8. Fashion Model Rain,
9. President Rain,
10. God's Child Two,
11.CEO Rain,
12 Author Rain
13. Bully Proof Rain
14.Rain Boy Fashion,
15. Football Team Rain,
16. Business Mogul Rain,
17. Pilot Rain,
18. Attorney Rain,
19. Rain's Children's Library,
20. Rain,
21. Philanthropist Rain,
22. Poet Rain
23.Rain Storybook Poem
24.Happy Mothers' Day.
25. Rain Magical Library
26. Rain Fields Incorporation
27.Rain Retirement Party,
28.Sir Knight Rain
29. Rain Vacation
30. Rain' Famous Friends

31. Firefighter Rain,
32. Prince Rain,
33. Musician Rain,
34. Fashion Designer Rain,
35. Cupcakes By Rain,
36. Astronaut Rain,
37. Photographer Rain,
38. Chef Rain,
39.Rain's Children's Book Museum,
40. Race Car Driver Rain,
41.The Rain Fields Children's book collection,
42.Atlantis Rain,
43.Sextillion Dollar Rain,
44.G.I.Rain,
45.Scientist Rain,
46. Gladiator Rain

Movies on Paper Studio **Fiction** Children's Book Collection.

1.BlueBerry Bedtime Story,
2. The Magic Cell Phone,
3.Red Rain Boots,
4. Bubble Bath Time,
5.Broccoli Meet Cheese,
6.Good Night Blanket,
7.The Lost Tooth,
8.Read Fairy,
9. Sitcoms On Paper, Episode 1
10.Episode 2

Movies on Paper Studio NonFiction Novels.

1.Movies On Paper Studio,
2. Dionne Fields Incorporation,
3. Honoring Colleges,
5. Documentary Of Real Champ,
6. Living For Today
7. September 11,
8. Sedreck Fields,
9.Greatness Endured 37 Losses,
10. Documentary Real Champ, 11. Sedreck Fields Scholarship Fund, 12. Ten Thousand Volunteer Hours, 13. No One Exempt From Hard Times, 14. National Book Signing, 15. Black History & Me, 16. 2012 By Dionne, 17. Theresita. 18. Unlimited God favor, 19. Black Movies On Paper, 20. Sedreck Fields Foundation, 21.Purpose & Reflections, 22. Behind Close Doors, 23.Facing Tomorrow 24. One Wish 25. History Maker Nominee 26. Dionne Fields Reality TV Show, 27. The Girl's Club, 28. Mascara, 29. The Director, 30. Waverly, 31.**Cancer Survival Museum**.32.

Movies on Paper Studio True - Crime Book Series.

1.The Untold Story,
2.Unpunished,
3. Whispering A Secret,
4.Pages Of Me Chapter One,
5. Pages Of Me Chapter Two,
6.Pages Of Me Chapter Three,
7. Pages Of Me Chapter Four,
8. Pages Of Me Chapter Five,
9. Pages Of Me Chapter Six,
10. Pages Of Me Chapter Seven,
11.

Movies on Paper Studio Ideas On Paper Book Series.

1.Re-designed Living Room Suite 2.Re-designed Lightweight Military Uniforms 3.Re-designed Toddler Strollers 4.Re-designed Ball Game Seats 5.Re-designed Lamps 6.Re-designed Bathroom Sets 7.Re-designed Business Chairs 8. Re-designed Car Seats, 9.Re-designed wall covers

A self help novel, to protect your loves from unfair health care and hospital treatments.

For years my mother had to endure unfair health care and hospital treatments.

First published in the United States of America in 2015
By Dionne Fields (Publisher) new hardcover edition.

Library Of Congress Cataloging-In-Publications Data
Fields, Dionne L.

[Movies On Paper Studio, Coming Soon To A Shelf Near You.]

Originally Published, 6331 Pleasant Ridge Road. Knoxville, Tennessee.37921

Library Of Congress Control Number:

ISBM 978-1507736128
ISBM 10-1507736126

http://www.onlineslibrary.webs.com

This novel was written and created By Dionne Fields

Printed in the United States of America January 26, 2015

Content Page

Movies On Paper Studio

Cancer survivor museum

Introduction by, Dionne Fields

Introduction page

Complete Book Title

Cancer survivor museum

Chapter 1

Cancer survivor museum for women diagnose with uterine cancer, ovarian cancer, cervical cancer, vaginal cancer and vulvar cancer.

This museum is in honor of my mother Theresita Fields.

She was diagnose with uterine cancer in 2012 and lost her fight just 10 days of her 64th birthday on October 26, 2012.

Chapter 2

This page you would see copies of legal documents and how one in the state of Tennessee, that tried to help my mother.

They did nothing to help her or to save her life.

The day my mother died, I lost my best friend and my mother all in the same day.

To help heal my broken heart, I'm telling the true story about my mother's untold story.

I want to help stop hospital negligence and wrongful deaths that happens every day in hospital.

This book is dedicated to my dear mom, with love always.

ISBN Page for Title : Cancer Survival Museum	
ISBN #:	**978-1507736128**
Content ID:	**1507736126**
Book Title:	Cancer Survival Museum

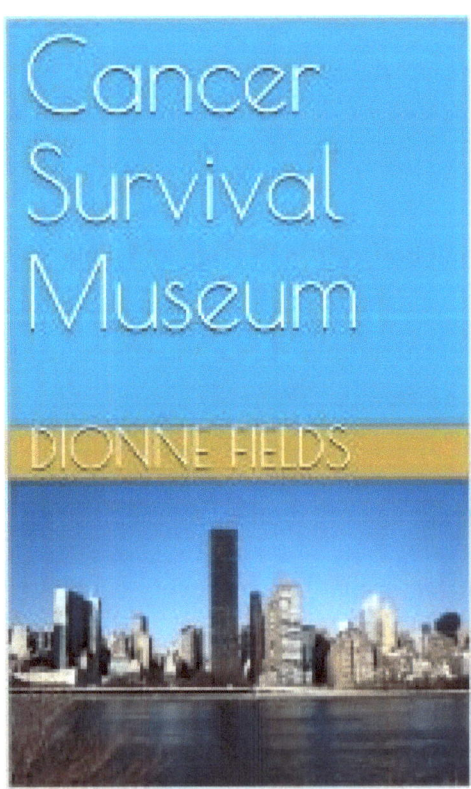

In loving memory of my beautiful mother.

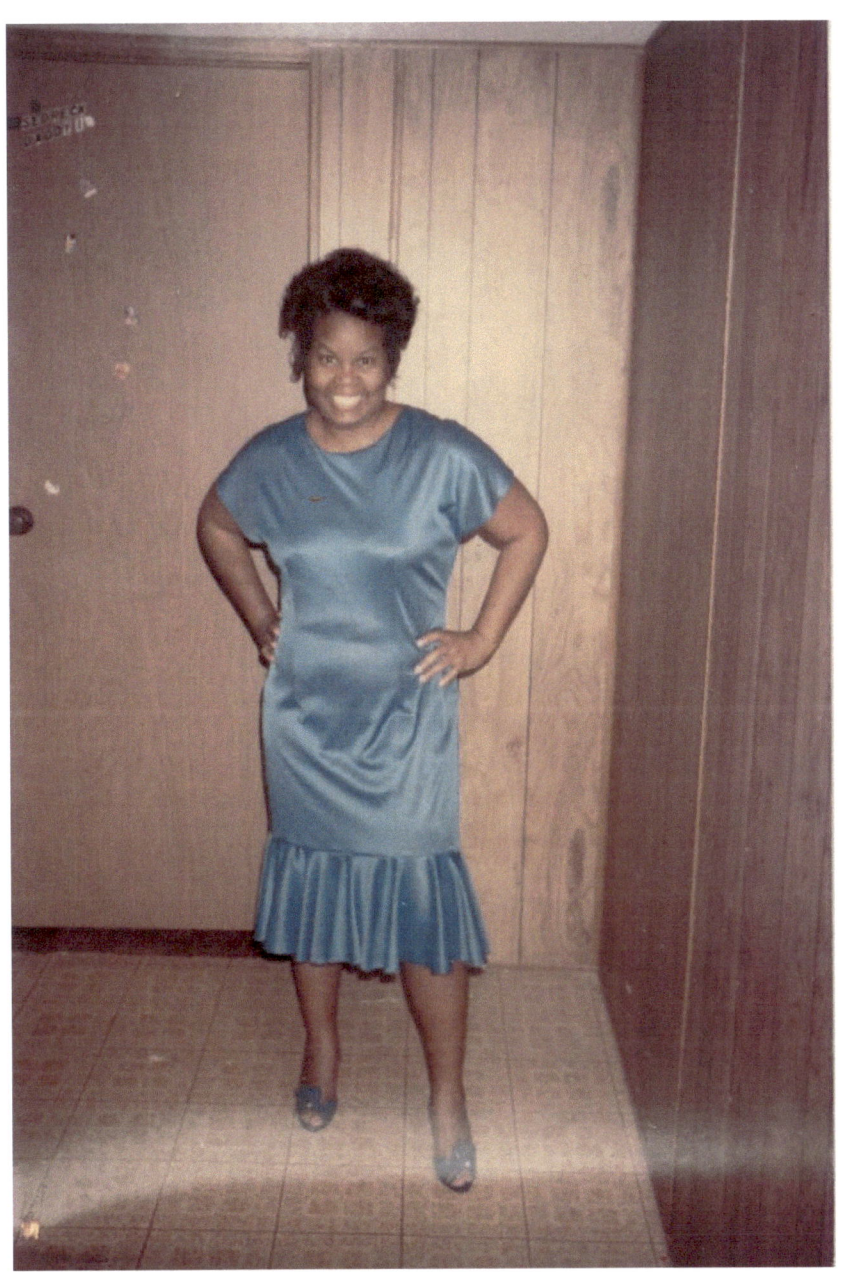

Theresita Fields
10-16-48 – 10-26-48

Chapter one

Title Page for: Cancer Survival Museum

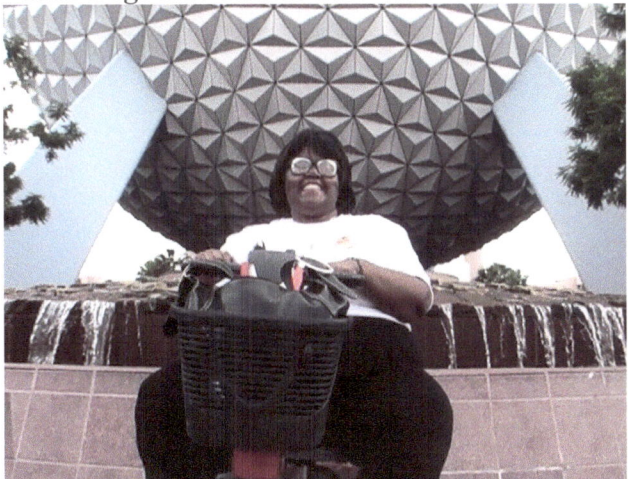

Cancer Survival Museum for Women.

Cancer survivor museum for women diagnose with uterine cancer, ovarian cancer, cervical cancer, vaginal cancer and vulvar cancer.

 This museum is in honor of my mother Theresita Fields.
She was diagnose with uterine cancer in 2012 and lost her fight just 10 days of her 64th birthday on October 26, 2012.

Thereista Fields 10-16-48- 10 26-12.

About uterine cancer
It's my goal to help woman fight Uterine Cancer.
To honor my mother's memory (Theresita Fields) 10-16-48 - 10-26-12.
And to raise funds for a new facility in Atlanta
near the Cancer Center of America.

Mission
My mother had Uterine Cancer. There was very little resource to help my mother, with her battle of Uterine Cancer. I want to help one million women, fight for the cure of uterine cancer. Uterine Cancer support group, survivor resources resource for, medicine, personal care items, wigs, food, ECT.

Biography
Read for the cure, I have books for sale to raise funds to
fight against Uterine Cancer.
I began writing novels after a career as a self-published author
and after publishing a dozen short stories.

Company Overview
My mission is to save lives and stop uterine cancer forever.
To also provide supportive services to woman impacted by a diagnosis of
uterine cancer. Your support will help give anyone facing
uterine cancer a place to turn for answers and help.

Description
The fight to cure uterine cancer and to raise funds for a new facility in Atlanta,
near the cancer center of America.
To provide the resource
and the support for women, who has been diagnosing with uterine cancer.

General Information
To provide assistance during the lowest point for women battling uterine cancer.
To partner with local community health charities to
offer women free to low cost yearly exams and pap smears.

How you can help
A benefit concert, local artist to donate live concert to raise funds, local radio thon
local radio station, walk to fight Uterine cancer, bake for the cure, local bakery donate
items for bake sale.

To honor your love one, in the cancer survival museum.

If you would like to honor your love one, by adding them to our cancer survival
museum you can honor them today with your contribution of $99 per person.

Today's special for a limited time is only $49 per person.

All the funds raise from your contribution will be use to purchase a building in the Atlanta, Georgia area.

You will receive an invitation to our grand opening once we purchase the cancer
survival museum.
Your love one name will all be feature inside the museum as well.

Theresita Fields 10-16-48 --- 10-26-12   Uterine Cancer   - $99
Your love one   Uterine cancer or ovarian cancer or cervical cancer-$49

http://theresit.webs.com/

I have found a list of services that could help you, if you have been diagnose with with uterine cancer, ovarian cancer, cervical cancer, vaginal cancer and vulvar cancer.

Academy of Oncology Nurse Navigators
aonnonline.org

the mission of the Academy of Oncology Nurse Navigators is to advance the role of patient navigation in cancer care and survivorship planning by providing a network for collaboration and development of best practices for the improvement of patient access to care and quality of life.

American Cancer Society
cancer.org

Provides comprehensive information for patients, family members and friends coping with cancer.

American Institute for Cancer Research
aicr.org
Advocates about the link between cancer and diet.

American Society of Clinical Oncology

asco.org

Aims to improve cancer care and prevention.

Be the Match
marrow.org

Helps people receive bone morrow transplants.

Cancer Care

cancercare.org

Offers free counseling, online support groups and educational workshops.

National Cancer Institute's Cancer Information Service

cancer.gov/aboutnci/cis

Helps people find local healthcare providers and treatment facilities.

National Cancer Institute's Clinical Trials

cancer.gov/clinicaltrials

Maintains a list of clinical trials.
Searchable by cancer type, stage, trial type and location.

National Coalition for Cancer Survivorship

canceradvocacy.org

Advocates for quality cancer care for all touched by cancer.

National Comprehensive Cancer Network

nccn.com
An alliance of cancer centers devoted to patient care, research and education.

Stupid Cancer

stupidcancer.org

A nonprofit organization that empowers young adults affected by cancer through innovative and award-winning programs and services.

Support for Patients and Families

Breakaway From Cancer

breakawayfromcancer.com

Offers people affected by cancer a broad range of support services complementing those provided by their healthcare professionals.

CancerCare

cancercare.org

Provides free, professional services for anyone affected by cancer including counseling, online support groups and free educational workshops.

Cancer.Net

cancer.net

Has oncologist-reviewed cancer information to help patients make informed healthcare decisions.

Cancer Support Community

cancersupportcommunity.org

Aims to ensure that all people impacted by cancer are empowered by knowledge, strengthened by action and sustained by community.

fertileHOPE

fertilehope.org

Provides reproductive information, support and hope to cancer patients whose medical treatments present the risk of infertility.

Living Beyond Breast Cancer

lbbc.org

Assists you whether you are newly diagnosed or in treatment for metastatic breast cancer.

National Lymphedema Network

lymphnet.org

Provides guidance on the prevention and management of lymphedema.

Patient Advocate Foundation

patientadvocate.org

Serves as a liaison between the patient and their insurer or creditors to resolve insurance or debt-crisis matters.

Sister Network

sisternetworkinc.org

This African American breast cancer survivorship organziation has outreach initiatives that promote the importance of breast health.

Someone With

someonewithbreastcancer.com

Leads you to the best products during and after treatment.

Women's Cancer Network

wcn.org

Offers patient support, education and information about new treatment options. Support for Caregivers

Caregiver Action Network

caregiveraction.org

The nation's leading family caregiving organization.

Savings and Financial Assistance

HealthMonitor Savings Dashboard

healthmonitor.com/AADE/savings.do

Savings for cancer patients.

American Cancer Society

cancer.org

For various types of financial help, search for "financial guidance for cancer survivors and their families."

CancerCare

cancercare.org

Offers assistance and resources for cancer-related costs.

Cancer Care Copay

cancercarecopay.org

Helps defray chemotherapy copays and cost of targeted treatment drugs.

Money Management International

moneymanagement.org

A full-service credit counseling agency.

Patient Advocate Foundation

patientadvocate.org

Serves as a liaison between the patient and insurer or creditors to resolve insurance and debt crisis matters.

Partnership for Prescription Assistance

pparx.org

Helps in getting prescription drugs even if you don't have coverage.

Scott Hamilton Cares

scottcares.org

Helps with chemo medications and treatment.

Survivorship A to Z

survivorshipatoz.org

Provides practical, financial and legal information after a life-changing diagnosis.
Free Gear

Cancer Fund of America, Inc.

cfoa.org/available_products.html

Provides toiletries and other everyday products.

Chemo Angels

chemoangels.net

Small gifts to people undergoing chemo.

Corporate Angel Network

www.corpangelnetwork.org

Provides free plane transportation for people going to and from certain recognized cancer treatment centers.

Good Wishes

goodwishesscarves.org

Provides free scarves and head wraps.

Hats Off to Chemo

hatsofftochemo.com

Click on "Request a Hat." Pick your style, then send a hat to yourself.

Heavenly Hats

heavenlyhats.com

Collects and distributes new hats to people who lose their hair due to cancer treatments.

The Lydia Project

thelydiaproject.org

Provides handmade tote bags, encouraging notes and prayers to women with cancer.

Reid Sleeve

reidsleeve.com

Peninsula Medical will send a medical alert bracelet to people with or at risk of lymphedema.

Click on "Free LE Alertband."

Services and Classes

Cleaning for a Reason

cleaningforareason.org

Links you with partnering housecleaning services in your area.

Look Good, Feel Better

lookgoodfeelbetter.org

Teaches beauty techniques to people with cancer to help them manage appearance-related side effects.

Yoga Bear

yogabear.org

Links you with partnering yoga studies offering free or donation only classes.
Click on "Find a free class."
Travel and Fun
Camp Mak-A-Dream *campdream.org*
Provides medically supervised retreats in Montana for children, young adults and families impacted by cancer.
Casting for Recovery *castingforrecovery.org*
Holds fly-fishing retreats for women who have or have had breast cancer.
Harmony Hill Retreat Center *harmonyhill.org*
Hosts one-day workshops and three-day retreats in Washington.
Little Pink Houses of Hope *littlepinkhousesofhope.org*
Provides weeklong beach retreats in the Carolinas for breast cancer patients and their families.

Uterine Cancer

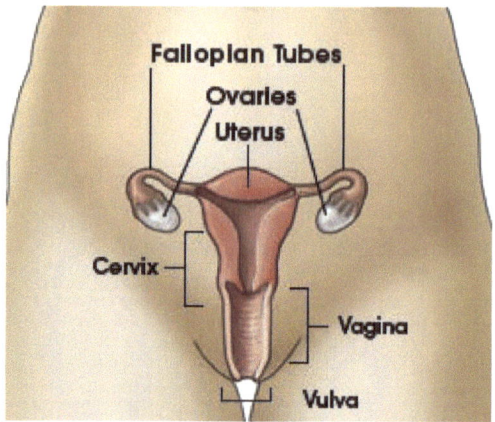

Cancer is a disease in which cells in the body grow out of control.
Cancer is always named for the part of the body where it starts, even if it spreads to other body parts later.

When cancer starts in the uterus, it is called **uterine cancer**.
The uterus is the pear-shaped organ in a woman's pelvis (the area below your stomach and in between your hip bones).

The uterus, also called the womb, is where the baby grows when a woman is pregnant. The most common type of uterine cancer is also called endometrial cancer because it forms in the lining of your uterus, called the endometrium.

When uterine cancer is found early, treatment is most effective.
Who Gets **Uterine Cancer?**

All women are at risk for uterine cancer, but the risk increases with age. Most uterine cancers are found in women who are going through or who have gone through menopause—the time of life when your menstrual periods stop.

Uterine cancer is the fourth most common cancer in women in the United States and the most commonly diagnosed gynecologic cancer.

Ovarian Cancer

When cancer starts in the ovaries, it is called **ovarian cancer**.

Women have two ovaries that are located in the pelvis, one on each side of the uterus. The ovaries make female hormones and produce eggs.
Ovarian cancer causes more deaths than any other cancer of the female reproductive system.
But when ovarian cancer is found in its early stages, treatment is most effective.

Ovarian cancer often causes signs and symptoms, so it is important to pay attention to your body and know what is normal for you.

Symptoms may be caused by something other than cancer, but the only way to know is to see your doctor, nurse, or other health care professional.

Who Gets **Ovarian Cancer?**

All women are at risk for ovarian cancer, but older women are more likely to get the disease than younger women.

About 90% of women who get ovarian cancer are older than 40 years of age, with the greatest number of cases occurring in women aged 60 years or older.

Each year, about 20,000 women in the United States get ovarian cancer.

Among women in the United States, ovarian cancer is the eighth most common cancer and the fifth leading cause of cancer death, after lung and bronchus, breast, colorectal, and pancreatic cancers.

Ovarian cancer causes more deaths than any other cancer of the female reproductive system, but it accounts for only about 3% of all cancers in women.

When ovarian cancer is found in its early stages, treatment is most effective.

Cervical Cancer

When cancer starts in the cervix, it is called **cervical cancer**.
The cervix is the lower, narrow end of the uterus.

The cervix connects the vagina (birth canal) to the upper part of the uterus. The uterus (or womb) is where a baby grows when a woman is pregnant.

Cervical cancer is highly preventable in most Western countries because screening tests and a vaccine to prevent HPV infections are available.

When cervical cancer is found early, it is highly treatable and associated with long survival and good quality of life.

Who Gets **Cervical Cancer?**

All women are at risk for cervical cancer. It occurs most often in women over age 30.
Each year, about 12,000 women in the United States get cervical cancer.

The human papillomavirus (HPV) is the main cause of cervical cancer. HPV is a common virus that is passed from one person to another during sex.

At least half of sexually active people will have HPV at some point in their lives, but few women will get cervical cancer.

Vaginal and Vulvar Cancers

When cancer starts in the vagina, it is called **vaginal cancer**.

The vagina, also called the birth canal, is the hollow, tube-like channel between the bottom of the uterus and the outside of the body.

When cancer starts in the vulva, it is called vulvar cancer.

The vulva is the outer part of the female genital organs.

It has two folds of skin, called the labia. Vulvar cancer most often occurs on the inner edges of the labia.

When vaginal and vulvar cancers are found early, treatment is most effective.

Who Gets **Vaginal and Vulvar Cancers?**

Vaginal and vulvar cancers are very rare.

While all women are at risk for these cancers, very few will get them.

 Together, they account for 6%–7% of all gynecologic cancers diagnosed in the U.S.

In 2010 the most recent year numbers are available

1,211 women in the United States were diagnosed with vaginal cancer.
423 women in the United States died from vaginal cancer.

4,305 women in the United States were diagnosed with vulvar cancer.
942 women in the United States died from vulvar cancer.

Friday Night Fights. *Monthly on the second Friday*

Local boxing gym in Atlanta Area (location announce soon)

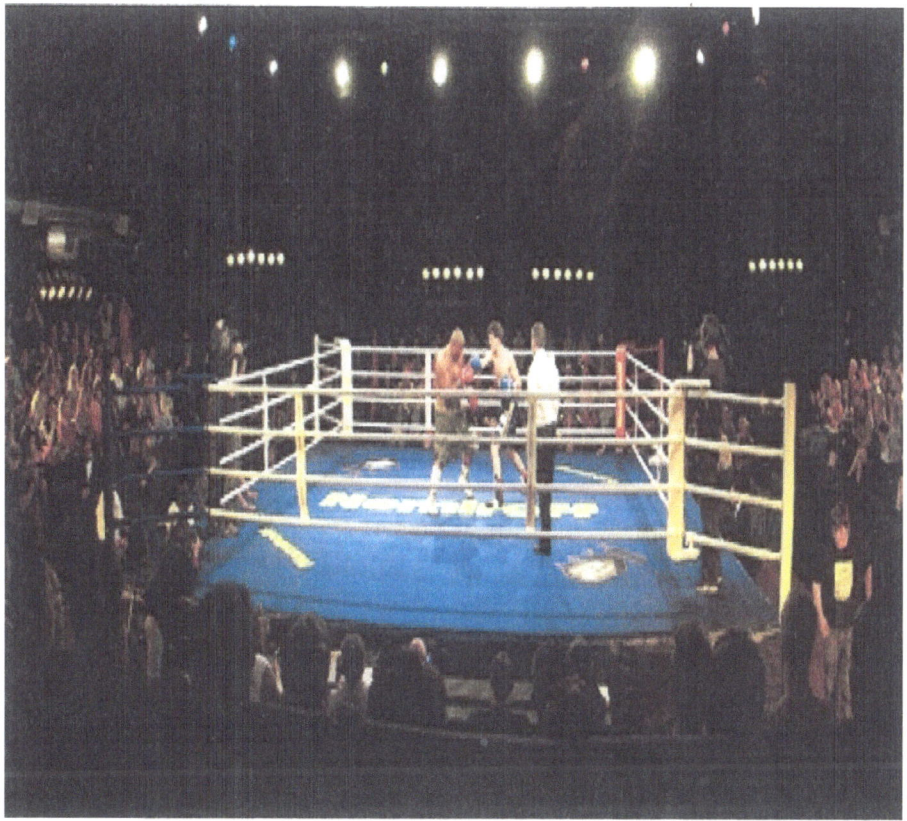

My mother was diagnosing with uterine cancer in 2012.
In her memory, we will be fighting for her to save lives and to end the disease of uterine
cancer.

The funds raised will be used to purchase a new facility for our organization.
To participate in this event, to fight against uterine cancer.

Team #1 pink with pink gloves is fighters.
Team #2 black with black gloves are uterine cancer.

The event is fighting against uterine cancer.3 rounds for 3 minutes each fight.

You may fight for a love one who has been diagnoses with uterine cancer.
(Fighters)And you can help find a cure for uterine cancer.

(Uterine cancer) Kids ages 5-10 cost to participate is only $10.00
each.
Boys against boys
Girls against girls

Fight time 5:00pm
Youth's ages 11-14 cost to participate is only $10.00 each.
Fight time 6:00pm
Teen's ages 14-17 cost to participate is only $10.00 each.
Fight time 7:00pm
Adults ages 18 and over cost to participate is only $20.00 each.
Group cost to fight a team of 6 is just $60.00.
Business cost to fight a team of 6 is just $60.00.
Fight time 8:00pm.
Register today, before all the seats and fights are sold out.
Tickets at the door to attend our fight night event.
Adult tickets just $10.00,
Kids tickets just $5.00
Free less than 3 years old.
Advance tickets purchase on line is only $7.00 Adults, (ages 18 and up)
Advance tickets purchase on line is only $5.00 kids (ages 5-17)
Advance tickets purchase online are only $30.00 per (Group and Business Teams)

You may purchase The Theresita Fields story her battle against Uterine Cancer today:

 http://www.amazon.com/Cancer-Survival-Museum-Dionne-Fields-ebook/dp/B00HOL38C0/ref=asap_bc?ie=UTF8

Just bring copy of book to the event to be autograph with your receipt.

And your admission is free!

Volunteers are needed to be ring girls.
Volunteers are needed to be referee.
Volunteers are needed to set up boxing ring.
Volunteers are needed to hand out flyer.
Volunteers are need to video record the event.
Volunteers are needed to take photos.
Business who would like to cater this event,
 Please email me today. Jesus1st2me@yahoo.com
The boxing gym location in Atlanta will be announced soon.
(TBA) Friday June 6, 2014
Sponsorship for this event is welcome.
Follow link below to register and purchase advance tickets.

EXAMPLE
Advance tickets for fighting on pink team.
Advance tickets for fighting on black team.
Advance ticket to attend fight night.
Thank you in advance for, helping us raises money for a new facility to help save lives.

Walk for the cure.

Monthly on the third Saturday, until July 13, 2015

Local bike trail and park in Atlanta Area (location announce soon)

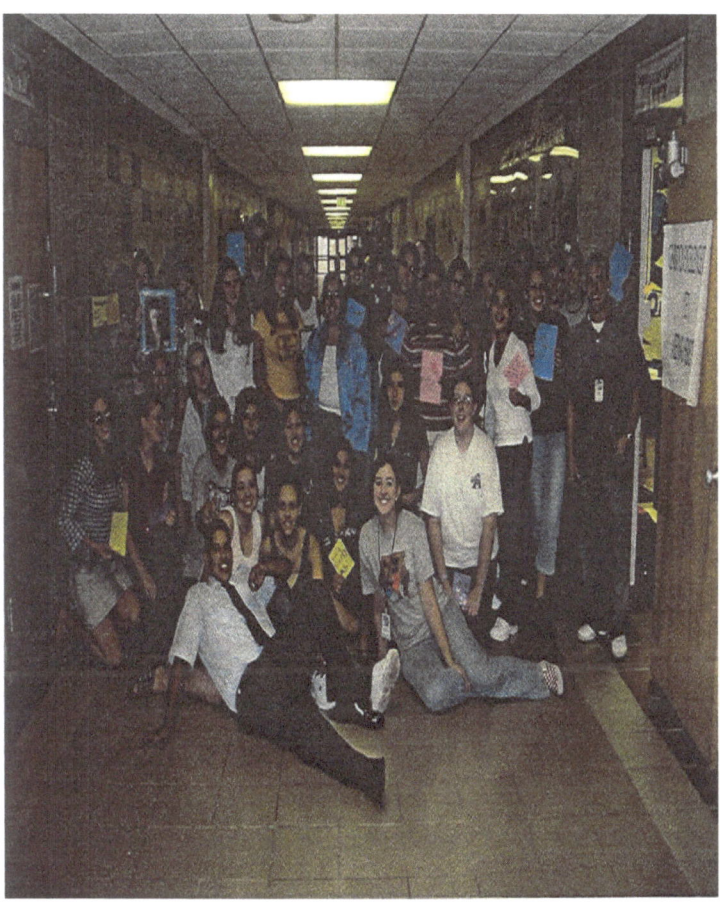

We will be walking at local bike trails and parks.
Our walk for the cure will also begin with a picnic.
Walk for a cure will be once a month on Saturday mornings.
Between 10 am and 12 noon.
Sponsors are welcome to support this event.
Volunteers are needed to hand out bottle water.
Volunteers are needed to set up pic nic tables.
Volunteers are needed to place pink and white balloons on bike trail and in the park.
To participate in this event is only $10 per person at the door.
And kids under the age of 18 are only $5 per child.
Mothers with strollers are $1.00.
Door prizes and free food will be given away.

Uterine Cancer Support Group.

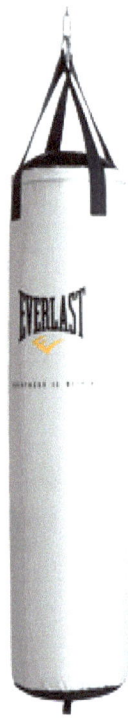

Monthly on the fourth Thursday, until July 13, 2015

The location will be at our new building, when we get the funds,

Uterine cancer survivals to come share their stories, to encourage other women during our weekly uterine cancer support group.

Thursdays 6-8pm a drawing for a gift basket at each meeting.

The community to donate non perishable items and can goods to our weekly food pantry, to help women diagnose with uterine cancer with children.

We also have a punching bag and gloves for women diagnose with uterine cancer.

To fight the bag to release stress and fears.

And to knock out uterine cancer.

To participate in knock out uterine cancer is only, $5.00 for every 10 minutes.

This is a wonderful event to raise funds and to have fun.

Music concert for the cure.

Monthly on the fourth Friday, until July 13, 2015

The park and event location will be announced soon.

A music concert for the cure.

Sponsors are welcome to help with this event.

Gospel music and praise and worship music is preferable.

Local artist or band to donate their talent to our monthly benefit concerts on Saturday, from 1-3pm

The cost is a donation of $3 per person.

And $5 dollar donation per family of 4 people.

Kids under 12 are free!!

Business to cater, this outdoor event are welcome.

Read for the cure

Read For A Cure Campaign.

Our goal is to sell one million books, to help one million women diagnose with Uterine Cancer.

For every book purchase, all proceeds will help save lives and raise funds for a new facility in Atlanta.

http://www.amazon.com/Cancer-Survival-Museum-Dionne-Fields-ebook/dp/B00HOL38C0/ref=asap_bc?ie=UTF8

To My Mother, With Love.

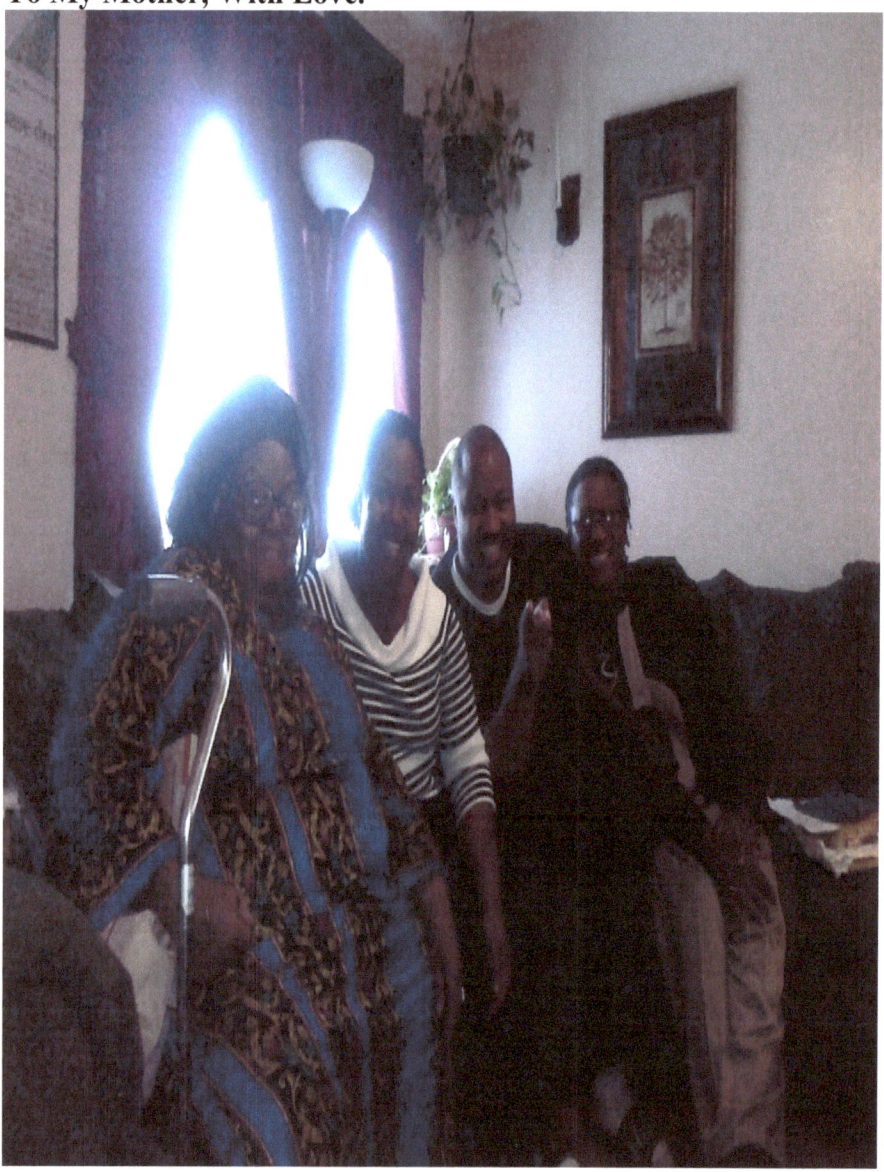

The fight against uterine cancer still continues.

Thanks mom, for always believing in me, and for buying me 1st novel.

Thanks mom for making me a better mother to my kids.

You are the reason I'm where I'm at today and thank you.

I love You Mom!!

You're Daughter (Dionne)

The Untold Story

A self help novel, to protect your loves from unfair health care and hospital treatments.

For years my mother had to endure unfair health care and hospital treatments.

I have filed over a dozen complaints, against the hospital and health care service for my mother.

No one would listen.

No one cared

No one did anything.

My name is Dionne Fields the daughter of Theresita Fields,

 I listen, I care and I'm doing something now.

My untold story

By Dionne Fields

A Daughter's Tears.

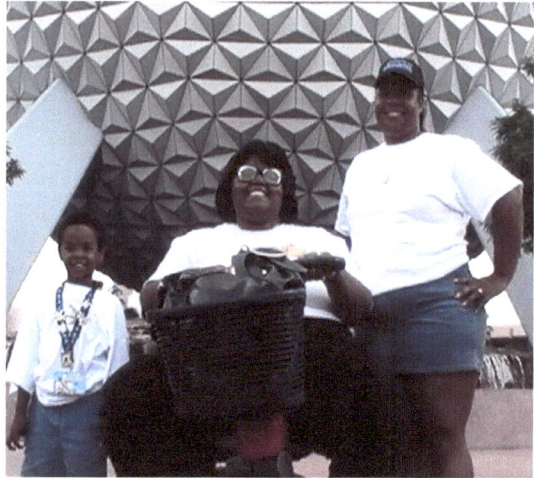

I started working on a personal journal the very day; my mother was diagnosing with uterine cancer mother's day 2012.Each day, that I visit her; I would take notes of her daily progress. Once she is in remission of her cancer, I will publish this journal into a self help novel at my online book store and library call Movies on Paper.

This new self help novel title **the untold story**, will help daughters of ages cope with having a parent, who is dying with any type of cancer. I have started an online cancer support group for daughters, who moms arc fighting Uterine Cancer. I pray that my experience with my mother, would help another daughter survives this painful, sleepless ,emotional , heart retching tragic , that I'm dealing with alone each and every day.

http://theresit.webs.com/

In my spare time when, I'm unable to sleep at night, I would work on my magazine called: **Cancer & Answers.** A health magazine, about cancer.

And also resource articles to help cancer patients, with help & support to make their fight against cancer much easier to fight. In my new magazine, I will feature the survival story of the month.

I believe God for the Funding to launch this new cancer magazine this year.

No one came to see my mother when she was diagnose, with stage 4 uterine cancers in May 2012.

No one help me bury my mother, when she died in October 2012.

During my painful emotional grieve, from the lost of my dear mother. I teach who my real family and friends where. The only person, who was there for me was God. Read for the cure campaign, it is my mission to help one million women, daignose with uterine cancer. 10% of all proceeds from this novel will benefit the Theresita Fields' Foundation.

My mother also needs her broken power chair replace, so she can get around and continue her daily radiation treatments .She also needs her mattress on her hospital bed replace, it is falling apart from every day wear and tear.

She has had the hardest time trying to get a work order for her broken power chair and replacement mattress for her bed.

It breaks my heart to see, mother denied of ever thing she needs to have some type of quality of life restored.

My mother suffers, so much from side effects from her radiation treatments and certain medications.

1. She suffers from dry mouth and throat, all foods and drinks taste like sand paper.
2. She takes daily nausea medicine, to keep from vomiting all day and night.
3. No control of her bladder, she wears depends adult diapers.

It's my goal to help my mother, regain her quality of life back.

In the near future, I Plan to move her back to Atlanta in the The Cancer center of America in Atlanta.

I believe this cancer treatment could help her in remission.

10% of all process from this book will be used, to purchase a building in Atlanta.

I will be opening a charity in my mother's honor, to help other women with uterine cancer and uterine cancer support.

I'm planning on purchasing a ford prius in the near future; it takes me 2 hours on the bus to get to my mother's house one way.

In a car I could take care of all my mother's daily needs in a couple of hours, but by bus it takes me days.

I'm so grateful to the dream foundation, for helping me with putting a smile on my mother's face.

This link is more information about my mother's charity.

http://theresit.webs.com/

My mother had so many obstacles in her life every sine, she was diagnose with uterine cancer mother day weekend 2012.

She has been suffering with pain from other health problems, before she was diagnose with cancer.

My mother suffers with chronic obstructive pulmonary disease and uses o2 dependency units at home, to help her breathe.

Wheel chair bound, her primary care doctor, refuse to do a work order for her wheel chair, so she can continue her daily radiation therapy.

1. Back pains, cause by denigrated disc disease.
2. Blockage in her upper colon, cause by not being able to make a bowel movement since April 2012.
3. Hemorrhoid the size of walnuts, 3 large one with split open sores. Doctors refuse to surgically remove them.
4. She is still passing kidney stones, after 3 kidney stone surgeries in the last six months.
5. High Blood pressure
6. Athirst in both knees
7. Poor speculation in both calves'.
8. My mom wears a nitro patch on her chest, for frequent chest pains.
9. She also uses an inhaler for her chronic bronchitis and shortness of breath.
10. She needs laser surgery on both eyes, so she can see where she is going.
11. Diverticulitis
12. Sleep Apnea
13. Chronic Obstructive Pulmonary Disease
14. Peptic ulcer disease (stomach cancer)

My mother can longer do things, she use to do for herself, due to her age and multiple health problems with her uterine cancer.

She can't bathe herself, fix her own meals, and clean her own home.

And pick up her own medication from the pharmacy and grocery shopping.

I help her each month with paying her bills and washing her clothes.

For months I saw my mother in out of Ft sanders hospital and traditional treatments at the Thompson survival center here in Knoxville TN.

My mother had many daily obstacles during her radiation treatments, like getting her insurance company blue care Medicaid to pay for all her medications, pain patch, and weekly pain medicine.

Also getting help at home, with a nurse to help her get around and someone to fix meals and light cleaning.

Dear, Grand mom

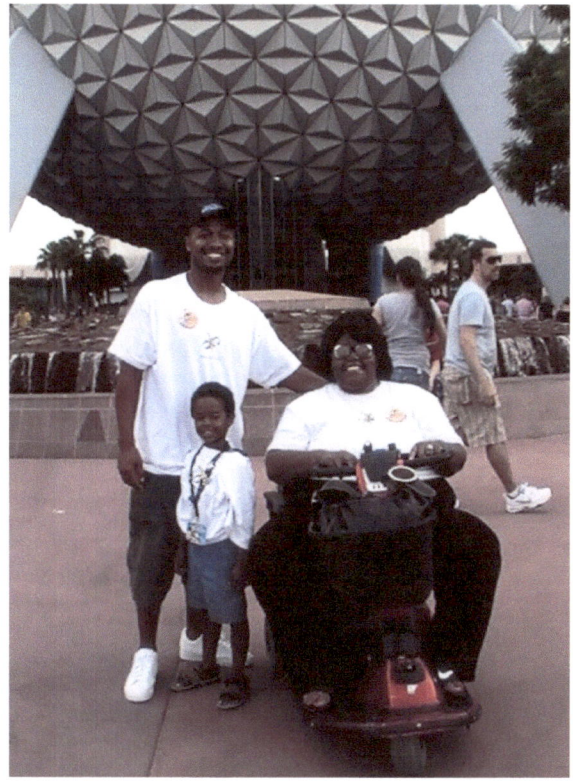

We love you, with all our heart you are the best grand mom in the world.

Thanks for making the sacrifice to spend with us during your illness of uterine cancer.

And most of all, thanks for taking us to Disney world to share in your dream.

We will miss you, and heaven now has the best grand mom in the world.

Love,

Diamond and Rain

On Thursday May 17, 2012

My mother's peptic ulcer disease (gastric ulcers) was no longer benign.

Her gastric ulcers developed into gastric malignancy (stomach cancer), she was never treated back in January 3, 2011 when it was in earlier stages.

Since no doctors had provided any type of treatment or monitors her gastric ulcer.

It had now spreading into her uterus and emergency Hysterectomy surgery had to be done on my mother the same day.

The doctor who did the surgery Dr Fields, told me that when she was diagnose with peptic ulcer disease (gastric ulcers) back in January 2011.

The hospital should have down exams, every time she complains about her virginal bleeding and severe abdominal pains.

Then they would have notice inflammation in her stomach.

And they could have treated her cancer in earlier stages.

I spoke to my mother doctor Dr Fields after he did my mother hysterectomy.

He said the pathologists after studying my mother's exam, they was not able to remove all the tumors. And at this point her cancer had reach stage four.

My mother's doctor told me he will start her on radiation therapy as soon as possible, to keep the cancer from spreading to her vital organs.

The doctor refers her to the oncology Dr. Tom Morgan of Fort sanders regional hospital.

The earliest the radiologist could see my mother was July 9, 2012 at 1:45pm, almost two months after her hysterectomy surgery that was done on May 17, 2012.

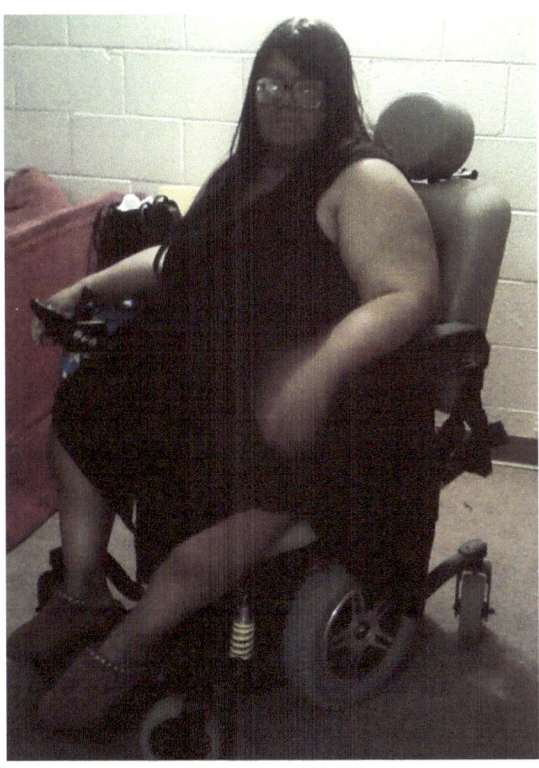

On Thursday October 4, 2012

My mother Theresita Fields went fort sanders regional hospital emergency room here in Knoxville TN.

My mother had been nausea, vomiting,constipation, and having acute chronic abdominal pain and chest pains.

The hospital sent my mother home to take miralax for constipation.

They failed to examine her abdominal bleeding and pains.

If they had took the time to do an exam on her abdomin, they would have notice that her cancer had spreaded with radaitional theraphy.

And the hospital would have started her on chemo right away.

My mother return back to the emergency room, days later with severe abdominal pains, nausea,vomiting,constipation.

The doctor notice that her cancer had spreaded,after doing a CT scan and MRI.

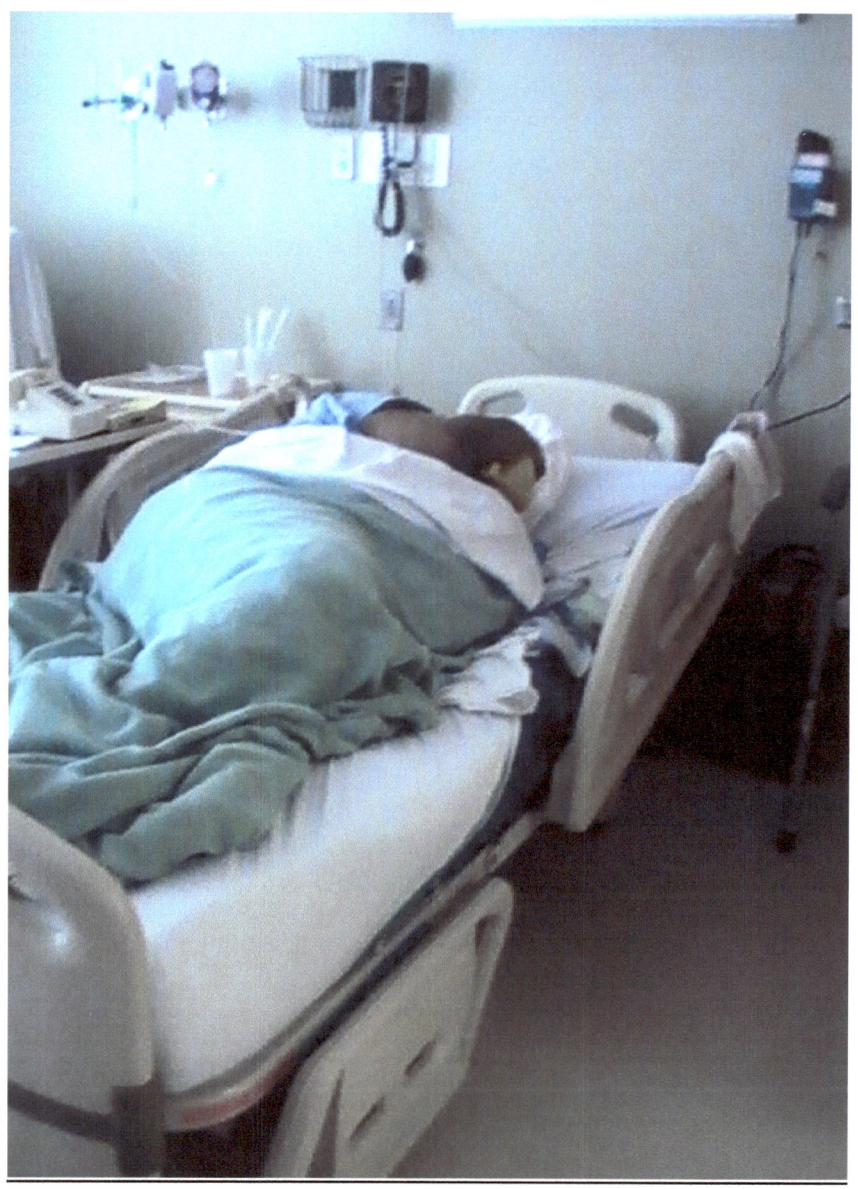

<u>Wednesday October 17, 2012</u>, when my mother was at home, she has to have oxygen all the time. She has been on Oxygen o2 dependency at home for a couple of years now. My mother was in so much pain and dehydration, that she was very weak. She couldn't stop from vomiting and she was very nausea. I ask the nurse could she give my mother something for nausea, to keep her from vomiting so much. She said she gave her something, earlier that day. I told the nurse it wasn't working, because my mother is still vomiting.

The nurse had an attitude and walk off, I kissed my mother and told her I was trying to get her located at the cancer center of America in Atlanta, so they could help her fight the spreading of her cancer and they would provide her with the best health care and treatments. I told my mother, I was still trying to get social security to approve her Medicare for the treatments at the cancer center of America in Atlanta.